AF260460

The Diabetic Diet Healthy Cooking Guide

50 recipes to cook as a family for any type of event

Roseann Smith

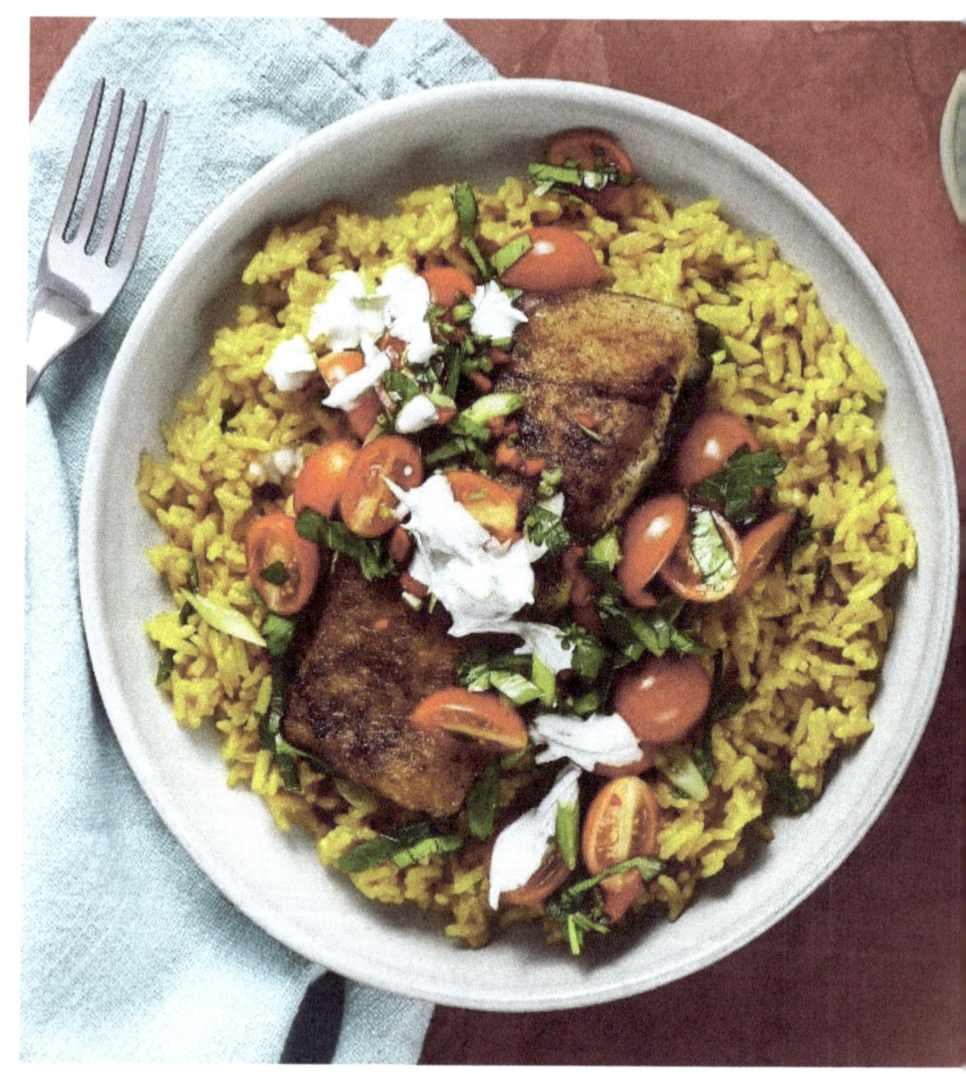

© Copyright 2021 - All rights reserved.

The content contained within this book may not be reproduced, duplicated or transmitted without direct written permission from the author or the publisher.

Under no circumstances will any blame or legal responsibility be held against the publisher, or author, for any damages, reparation, or monetary loss due to the information contained within this book. Either directly or indirectly.

Legal Notice:

This book is copyright protected. This book is only for personal use. You cannot amend, distribute, sell, use, quote or paraphrase any part, or the content within this book, without the consent of the author or publisher.

Disclaimer Notice:

Please note the information contained within this document is for educational and entertainment purposes only. All effort has been executed to present accurate, up to date, and reliable, complete information. No warranties of any kind are declared or implied. Readers acknowledge that the author is not engaging in the rendering of legal, financial, medical or professional advice. The content within this book has been derived from various sources. Please consult a licensed professional before attempting any techniques outlined in this book.

By reading this document, the reader agrees that under no circumstances is the author responsible for any losses, direct or indirect, which are incurred as a result of the use of information contained within this document, including, but not limited to, — errors, omissions, or inaccuracies.

Table of Contents

Shrimp Salad

Servings: 6

Cooking Time: 4 Minutes

Ingredients:

- For Salad:
- 1 pound shrimp, peeled and deveined
- Salt and ground black pepper, as required
- 1 teaspoon olive oil
- 1½ cups carrots, peeled and julienned
- 1½ cups red cabbage, shredded
- 1½ cup cucumber, julienned
- 5 cups fresh baby arugula
- ¼ cup fresh basil, chopped
- ¼ cup fresh cilantro, chopped
- 4 cups lettuce, torn
- ¼ cup almonds, chopped
- For Dressing:
- 2 tablespoons natural almond butter
- 1 garlic clove, crushed

- 1 tablespoon fresh cilantro, chopped
- 1 tablespoon fresh lime juice
- 1 tablespoon unsweetened applesauce
- 2 teaspoons balsamic vinegar
- ½ teaspoon cayenne pepper
- Salt, as required
- 1 tablespoon water
- 1/3 cup olive oil

Directions:

1. Slowly, add the oil, beating continuously until smooth.
2. For salad: in a bowl, add shrimp, salt, black pepper and oil and toss to coat well.
3. Heat a skillet over medium-high heat and cook the shrimp for about 2 minutes per side.
4. Remove from the heat and set aside to cool.
5. In a large bowl, add the shrimp, vegetables and mix well.
6. For dressing: in a bowl, add all ingredients except oil and beat until well combined.
7. Place the dressing over shrimp mixture and gently, toss to coat well.

8. Serve immediately.

9. Meal Prep Tip: Divide dressing in 6 large mason jars evenly. Place the remaining ingredients in the layers of carrots, followed by cabbage, cucumber, arugula, basil, cilantro, shrimp, lettuce and almonds. Cover each jar with the lid tightly and refrigerate for about 1 day. Shake the jars well just before serving.

Nutrition Info: Calories 274 Total Fat 17.7 g Saturated Fat 2.4 g Cholesterol 159 mg Total Carbs 10 g Sugar 3.8 g Fiber 2.9 g Sodium 242 mg Potassium 481 mg Protein 20.5 g

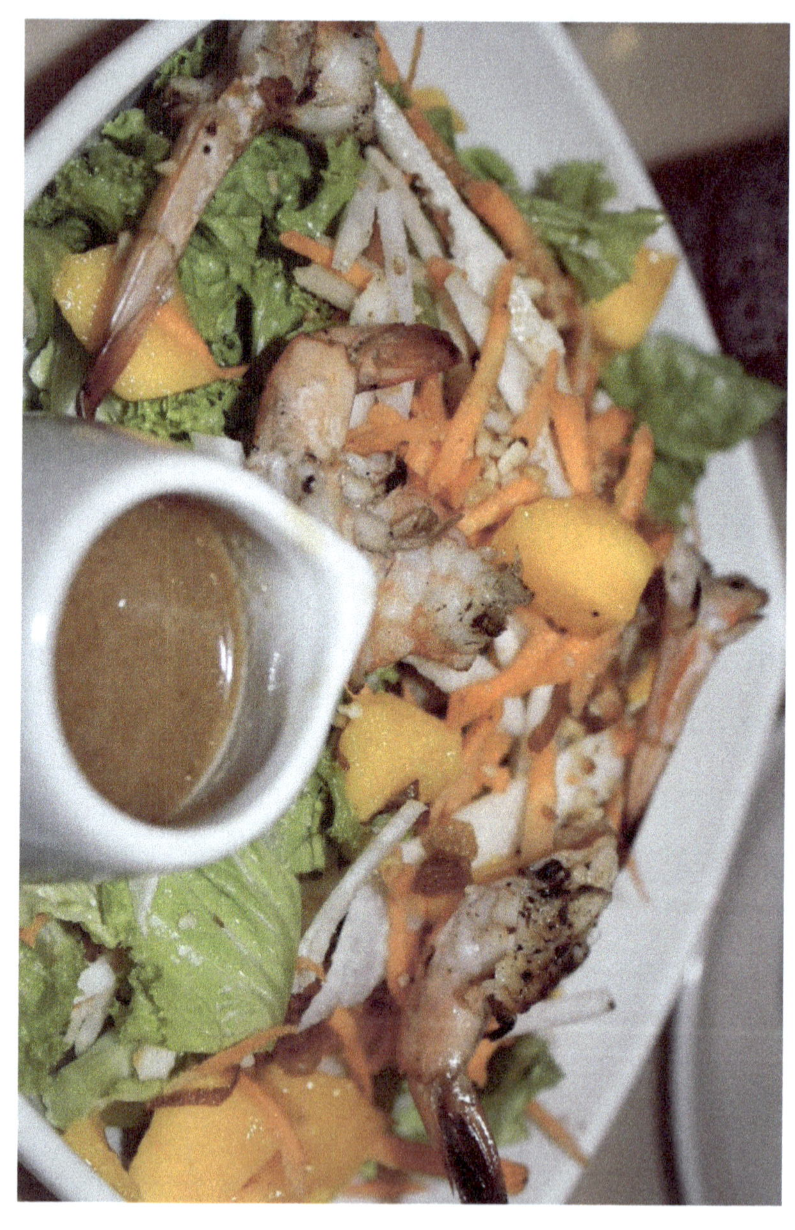

Grilled Herbed Salmon With Raspberry Sauce & Cucumber Dill Dip

Servings: 4

Cooking Time: 30 Minutes

Ingredients:

- 3 salmon fillets
- 1 tablespoon olive oil
- Salt and pepper to taste
- 1 teaspoon fresh sage, chopped
- 1 tablespoon fresh parsley, chopped
- 2 tablespoons apple juice
- 1 cup raspberries
- 1 teaspoon Worcestershire sauce
- 1 cup cucumber, chopped
- 2 tablespoons light mayonnaise
- ½ teaspoon dried dill

Directions:

1. Coat the salmon fillets with oil.
2. Season with salt, pepper, sage and parsley.
3. Cover the salmon with foil.
4. Grill for 20 minutes or until fish is flaky.
5. While waiting, mix the apple juice, raspberries and Worcestershire sauce.
6. Pour the mixture into a saucepan over medium heat.
7. Bring to a boil and then simmer for 8 minutes.
8. In another bowl, mix the rest of the ingredients.
9. Serve salmon with raspberry sauce and cucumber dip.

Nutrition Info: Calories 301 Fat 27.2 g Carbohydrates 13.6 g Protein 4.9 g Cholesterol 33 mg

Cajun Shrimp & Roasted Vegetables

Servings: 4

Cooking Time: 15 Minutes

Ingredients:

- 1 lb. large shrimp, peeled and deveined
- 2 zucchinis, sliced
- 2 yellow squash, sliced
- ½ bunch asparagus, cut into thirds
- 2 red bell pepper, cut into chunks
- What you'll need from store cupboard:
- 2 tbsp. olive oil
- 2 tbsp. Cajun Seasoning
- Salt & pepper, to taste

Directions:

1. Heat oven to 400 degrees.

2. Combine shrimp and vegetables in a large bowl. Add oil and seasoning and toss to coat.

3. Spread evenly in a large baking sheet and bake 15-20 minutes, or until vegetables are tender. Serve.

Nutrition Info: Calories 251 Total Carbs 13g Net Carbs 9g Protein 30g Fat 9g Sugar 6g Fiber 4g

Parmesan Herb Fish

Servings: 4

Cooking Time: 15 Minutes

Ingredients:

- 16 oz. tilapia fillets
- 1/3 cup almonds, sliced and chopped
- ½ teaspoon parsley, chopped
- ¼ cup dry bread crumbs
- What you will need from the store cupboard:
- ½ teaspoon garlic powder
- ¼ teaspoon black pepper, ground
- ½ teaspoon paprika
- 3 tablespoons Parmesan cheese, grated
- Olive oil

Directions:

1. Preheat your oven to 350 °F.

2. Mix the bread crumbs, almonds, seasonings and Parmesan cheese in a dish.

3. Brush oil lightly on the fish.

4. Coat the almond mix evenly.

5. Now keep the fish on a greased foil-lined baking pan.

6. Bake for 10-12 minutes. The fish should flake easily with your fork.

Nutrition Info: Calories 225, Carbohydrates 7g, Fiber 1g, Cholesterol 57mg, Total Fat 9g, Protein 29g, Sodium 202mg

Lemony Salmon

Servings: 3

Cooking Time: 3 Minutes

Ingredients:

- 1 pound salmon fillet, cut into 3 pieces
- 3 teaspoons fresh dill, chopped
- 5 tablespoons fresh lemon juice, divided
- Salt and ground black pepper, as required

Directions:

1. Arrange a steamer trivet in Instant Pot and pour ¼ cup of lemon juice.
2. Season the salmon with salt and black pepper evenly.
3. Place the salmon pieces on top of trivet, skin side down and drizzle with remaining lemon juice.
4. Now, sprinkle the salmon pieces with dill evenly.

5. Close the lid and place the pressure valve to "Seal" position.

6. Press "Steam" and use the default time of 3 minutes.

7. Press "Cancel" and allow a "Natural" release.

8. Open the lid and serve hot.

Nutrition Info: Calories: 20 Fats: 9.6g, Carbs: 1.1g, Sugar: 0.5g, Proteins: 29.7g, Sodium: 74mg

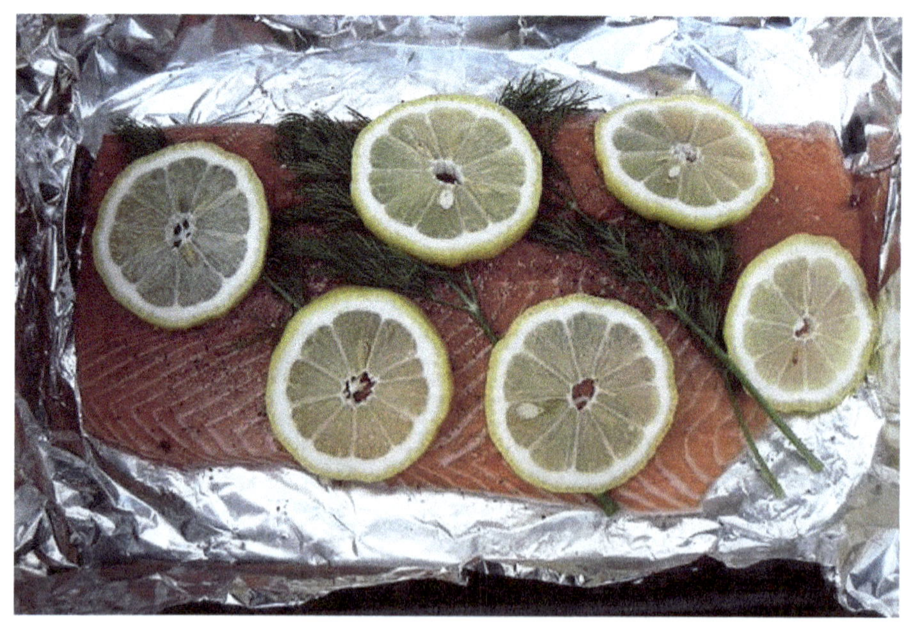

Herring & Veggies Soup

Servings: 5

Cooking Time: 25 Minutes

Ingredients:

- 2 tablespoons olive oil
- 1 shallot, chopped
- 2 small garlic cloves, minced
- 1 jalapeño pepper, chopped
- 1 head cabbage, chopped
- 1 small red bell pepper, seeded and chopped finely
- 1 small yellow bell pepper, seeded and chopped finely
- 5 cups low-sodium chicken broth
- 2 (4-ounce) boneless herring fillets, cubed
- ¼ cup fresh cilantro, minced
- 2 tablespoons fresh lemon juice
- Ground black pepper, as required
- 2 scallions, chopped

Directions:

1. In a large soup pan, heat the oil over medium heat and sauté shallot and garlic for 2-3 minutes.
2. Add the cabbage and bell peppers and sauté for about 3-4 minutes.
3. Add the broth and bring to a boil over high heat.
4. Now, reduce the heat to medium-low and simmer for about 10 minutes.
5. Add the herring cubes and cook for about 5-6 minutes.
6. Stir in the cilantro, lemon juice, salt and black pepper and cook for about 1-2 minutes.
7. Serve hot with the topping of scallion.
8. Meal Prep Tip: Transfer the soup into a large bowl and set aside to cool. Divide the soup into 5 containers evenly. Cover the containers and refrigerate for 1-2 days. Reheat in the microwave before serving.

Nutrition Info: Calories 215 Total Fat 11.2g Saturated Fat 2.1 g Cholesterol 35 mg Total Carbs 14.7 g Sugar 7 g Fiber 4.5 g Sodium 152 mg Potassium 574 mg Protein 15.1 g

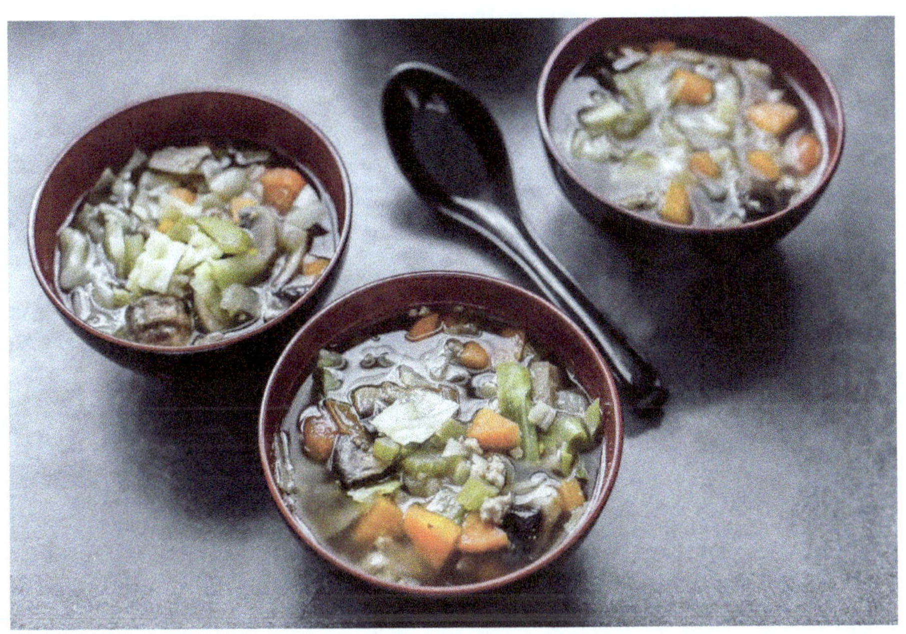

Garlicky Clams

Servings: 4

Cooking Time: 5 Minutes

Ingredients:

- 3 lbs clams, clean
- 4 garlic cloves
- 1/4 cup olive oil
- 1/2 cup fresh lemon juice
- 1 cup white wine
- Pepper
- Salt

Directions:

1. Add oil into the inner pot of instant pot and set the pot on sauté mode.
2. Add garlic and sauté for 1 minute.
3. Add wine and cook for 2 minutes.
4. Add remaining ingredients and stir well.
5. Seal pot with lid and cook on high for 2 minutes.

6.   Once done, allow to release pressure naturally. Remove lid.

7.   Serve and enjoy.

Nutrition Info: Calories 332 Fat 13.5 g Carbohydrates 40.5 g Sugar 12.4 g Protein 2.5 g Cholesterol 0 mg

Tuna Salad

Servings: 2

Ingredients:

- 2 (5-ounce) cans water packed tuna, drained
- 2 tablespoons fat-free plain Greek yogurt
- Salt and ground black pepper, as required
- 2 medium carrots, peeled and shredded
- 2 apples, cored and chopped
- 2 cups fresh spinach, torn

Directions:

1. In a large bowl, add the tuna, yogurt, salt and black pepper and gently, stir to combine.
2. Add the carrots and apples and stir to combine.
3. Serve immediately.
4. Meal Prep Tip: Divide tuna mixture in 2 mason jars evenly. Place the remaining ingredients in the layers of, carrots, apples and spinach. Cover each jar with the lid

tightly and refrigerate for about 1 day. Shake the jars well just before serving.

Nutrition Info: Calories 306 Total Fat 1.8g Saturated Fat 0 g Cholesterol 63 mg Total Carbs 38 g Sugar 26 g Fiber 7.6 g Sodium 324 mg Potassium 602 mg Protein 35.8 g

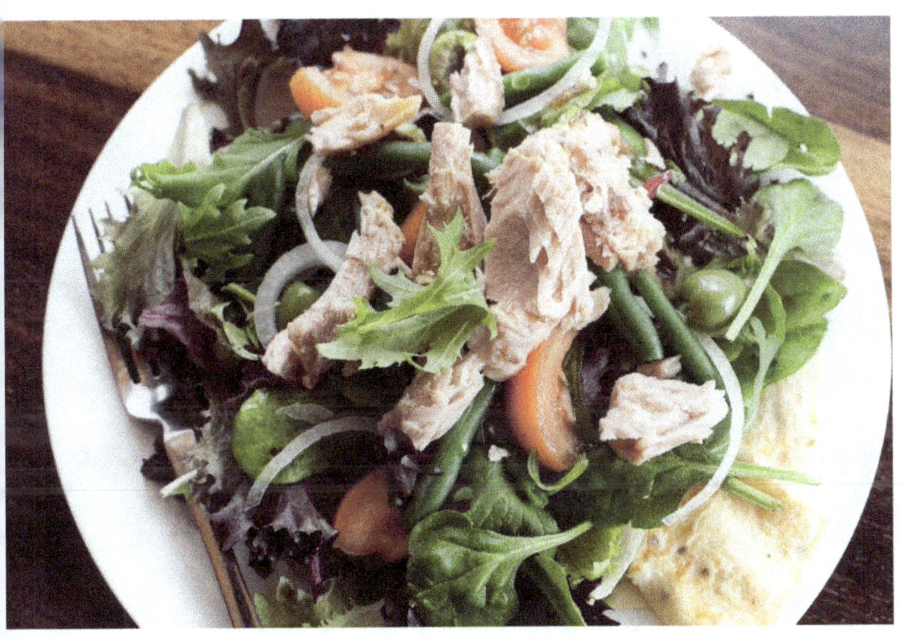

Grilled Tuna Salad

Servings: 4

Cooking Time: 15 Minutes

Ingredients:

- 4 oz. tuna fish, 4 steaks
- ¾ lb. red potatoes, diced
- ½ lb. green beans, trimmed
- 16 kalamata olives, chopped
- 4 cups of baby spinach leaves
- What you will need from the store cupboard:
- 2 tablespoons canola oil
- 2 tablespoons red wine vinegar
- 1/8 teaspoon salt
- 1 tablespoon water
- 1/8 teaspoon red pepper flakes

Directions:

1. Steam the green beans and potatoes to make them tender.
2. Drain, rinse to shake off the excess water.
3. Bring together the vinaigrette ingredients in your jar while the vegetables are cooking. Close the lid and shake well. Everything should blend well.
4. Brush the vinaigrette over your fish.
5. Coat canola oil on your pan. Heat over medium temperature.
6. Grill each side of the tuna for 3 minutes.
7. Now divide the greens on your serving plates.
8. Arrange the green beans, olives, and potatoes over the greens.
9. Drizzle the vinaigrette on the salad. Top with tuna.

Nutrition Info: Calories 345, Carbohydrates 26g, Fiber 5g, Cholesterol 40mg, Total Fat 14g, Protein 29g, Sodium 280mg

Mediterranean Fish Fillets

Servings: 4

Cooking Time: 3 Minutes

Ingredients:

- 4 cod fillets
- 1 lb grape tomatoes, halved
- 1 cup olives, pitted and sliced
- 2 tbsp capers
- 1 tsp dried thyme
- 2 tbsp olive oil
- 1 tsp garlic, minced
- Pepper
- Salt

Directions:

1. Pour 1 cup water into the instant pot then place steamer rack in the pot.
2. Spray heat-safe baking dish with cooking spray.
3. Add half grape tomatoes into the dish and season with pepper and salt.
4. Arrange fish fillets on top of cherry tomatoes. Drizzle with oil and season with garlic, thyme, capers, pepper, and salt.
5. Spread olives and remaining grape tomatoes on top of fish fillets.
6. Place dish on top of steamer rack in the pot.
7. Seal pot with a lid and select manual and cook on high for 3 minutes.
8. Once done, release pressure using quick release. Remove lid.
9. Serve and enjoy.

Nutrition Info: Calories 212 Fat 11.9 g Carbohydrates 7.1 g Sugar 3 g Protein 21.4 g Cholesterol 55 mg

Herbed Salmon

Servings: 4

Cooking Time: 3 Minutes

Ingredients:

- 4 (4-ounce) salmon fillets
- ¼ cup olive oil
- 2 tablespoons fresh lemon juice
- 1 garlic clove, minced
- ¼ teaspoon dried oregano
- Salt and ground black pepper, as required
- 4 fresh rosemary sprigs
- 4 lemon slices

Directions:

1. For dressing: in a large bowl, add oil, lemon juice, garlic, oregano, salt and black pepper and beat until well co combined.
2. Arrange a steamer trivet in the Instant Pot and pour 11/2 cups of water in Instant Pot.

3. Place the salmon fillets on top of trivet in a single layer and top with dressing.

4. Arrange 1 rosemary sprig and 1 lemon slice over each fillet.

5. Close the lid and place the pressure valve to "Seal" position.

6. Press "Steam" and just use the default time of 3 minutes.

7. Press "Cancel" and carefully allow a "Quick" release.

8. Open the lid and serve hot.

Nutrition Info: Calories 262, Fats 17g, Carbs 0.7g, Sugar 0.2g, Proteins 22.1g, Sodium 91mg

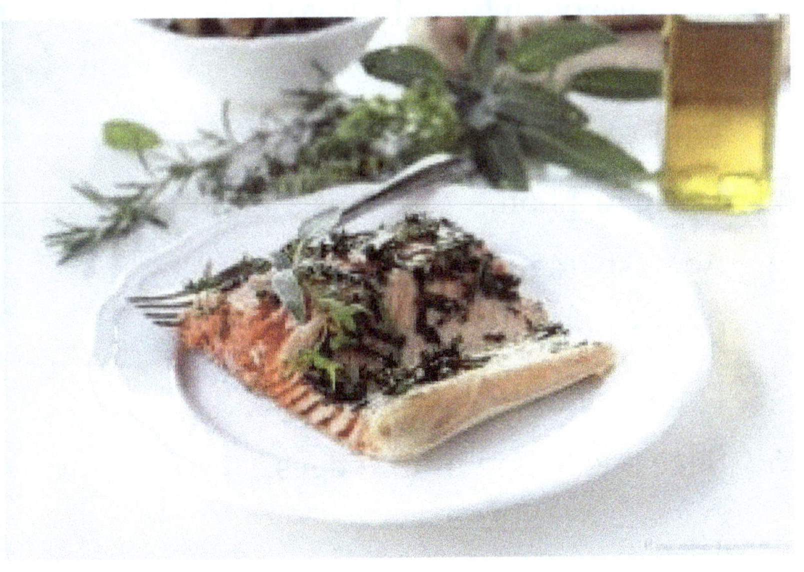

Tarragon Scallops

Servings: 4

Cooking Time: 15 Minutes

Ingredients:

- 1 cup water
- 1 lb. asparagus spears, trimmed
- 2 lemons
- 1 ¼ lb. scallops
- Salt and pepper to taste
- 1 tablespoon olive oil
- 1 tablespoon fresh tarragon, chopped

Directions:

1. Pour water into a pot.
2. Bring to a boil.
3. Add asparagus spears.
4. Cover and cook for 5 minutes.
5. Drain and transfer to a plate.
6. Slice one lemon into wedges.

7. Squeeze juice and shred zest from the remaining lemon.

8. Season the scallops with salt and pepper.

9. Put a pan over medium heat.

10. Add oil to the pan.

11. Cook the scallops until golden brown.

12. Transfer to the same plate, putting scallops beside the asparagus.

13. Add lemon zest, juice and tarragon to the pan.

14. Cook for 1 minute.

15. Drizzle tarragon sauce over the scallops and asparagus.

Nutrition Info: Calories 250 g Fat 10 g Carbohydrates 30 g Protein 15 g Cholesterol 24 mg

Sardine Curry

Servings: 2

Cooking Time: 35 Minutes

Ingredients:

- 5 tins of sardines in tomato
- 1lb chopped vegetables
- 1 cup low sodium fish broth
- 3tbsp curry paste

Directions:

1. Mix all the ingredients in your Instant Pot.
2. Cook on Stew for 35 minutes.
3. Release the pressure naturally.

Nutrition Info: Calories 320; Carbs 8; Sugar 2; Fat 16; Protein GL 3

Grilled Salmon With Ginger Sauce

Servings: 4

Cooking Time: 8 Minutes

Ingredients:

- 1 tablespoon toasted sesame oil
- 1 tablespoon fresh cilantro, chopped
- 1 tablespoon lime juice
- 1 teaspoon fish sauce
- 1 clove garlic, mashed
- 1 teaspoon fresh ginger, grated
- 1 teaspoon jalapeño pepper, minced
- 4 salmon fillets
- 1 tablespoon olive oil
- Salt and pepper to taste

Directions:

1. In a bowl, mix the sesame oil, cilantro, lime juice, fish sauce, garlic, ginger and jalapeño pepper.
2. Preheat your grill.
3. Brush oil on salmon.
4. Season both sides with salt and pepper.
5. Grill salmon for 6 to 8 minutes, turning once or twice.
6. Take 1 tablespoon from the oil mixture.
7. Brush this on the salmon while grilling.
8. Serve grilled salmon with the remaining sauce.

Nutrition Info: Calories 204 Total Fat 11 g Saturated Fat 2 g Cholesterol 53 mg Sodium 320 mg Total Carbohydrate 2 g Dietary Fiber 0 g Total Sugars 2 g Protein 23 g Potassium 437 mg

Shrimp With Broccoli

Servings: 6

Cooking Time: 12 Minutes

Ingredients:

- 2 tablespoons olive oil, divided
- 4 cups broccoli, chopped
- 2-3 tablespoons filtered water
- 1½ pounds large shrimp, peeled and deveined
- 2 garlic cloves, minced
- 1 (1-inch) piece fresh ginger, minced
- Salt and ground black pepper, as required

Directions:

1. In a large skillet, heat 1 tablespoon of oil over medium-high heat and cook the broccoli for about 1-2 minutes stirring continuously.

2. Stir in the water and cook, covered for about 3-4 minutes, stirring occasionally.

3. With a spoon, push the broccoli to side of the pan.

4. Add the remaining oil and let it heat.

5. Add the shrimp and cook for about 1-2 minutes, tossing occasionally.

6. Add the remaining ingredients and sauté for about 2-3 minutes.

7. Serve hot.

8. Meal Prep Tip: Transfer the shrimp mixture into a large bowl and set aside to cool. Divide the shrimp mixture into 6 containers evenly. Cover the containers and refrigerate for 1 day. Reheat in the microwave before serving.

Nutrition Info: Calories 197 Total Fat 6.8 g Saturated Fat 1.3 g Cholesterol 239 mg Total Carbs 6.1 g Sugar 1.1 g Fiber 1.6 g Sodium 324 mg Potassium 389 mg Protein 27.6 g

Citrus Salmon

Servings: 4

Cooking Time: 7 Minutes

Ingredients:

- 4 (4-ounce) salmon fillets
- 1 cup low-sodium chicken broth
- 1 teaspoon fresh ginger, minced
- 2 teaspoons fresh orange zest, grated finely
- 3 tablespoons fresh orange juice
- 1 tablespoon olive oil
- Ground black pepper, as required

Directions:

1. In Instant Pot, add all ingredients and mix.
2. Close the lid and place the pressure valve to "Seal" position.
3. Press "Manual" and cook under "High Pressure" for about 7 minutes.
4. Press "Cancel" and allow a "Natural" release.

5. Open the lid and serve the salmon fillets with the topping of cooking sauce.

Nutrition Info: Calories 190, Fats 10.5g, Carbs 1.8g, Sugar 1g, Proteins 22. Sodium 68mg

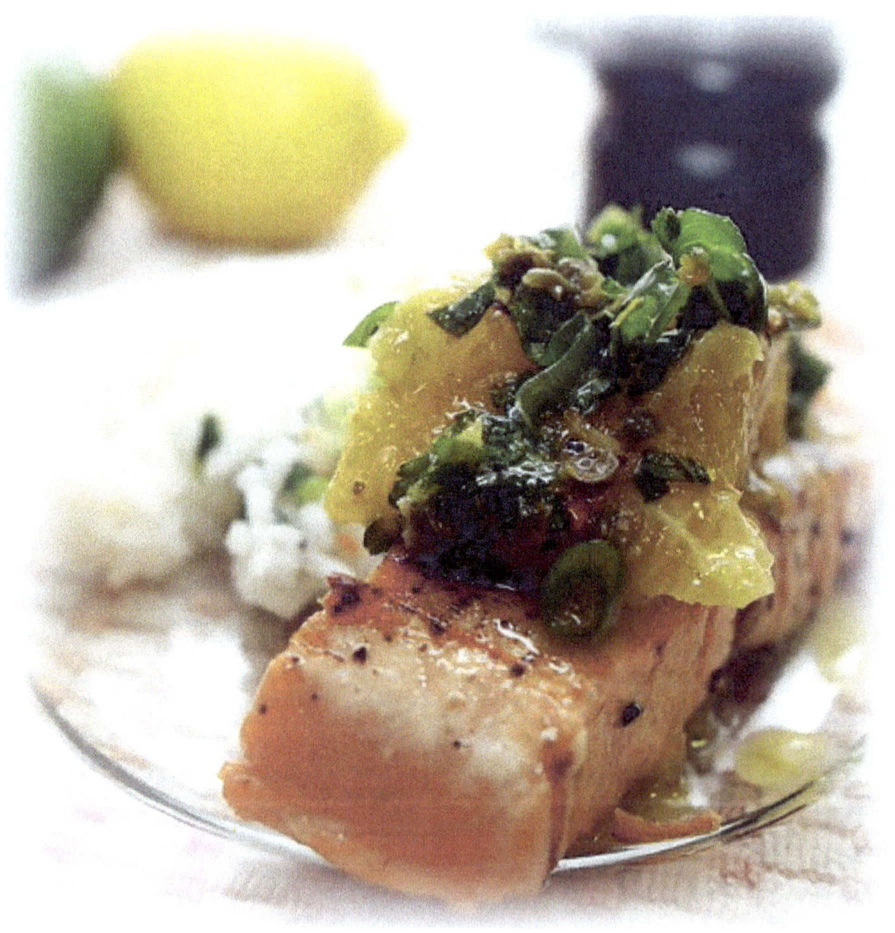

Salmon In Green Sauce

Servings: 4

Cooking Time: 12 Minutes

Ingredients:

- 4 (6-ounce) salmon fillets
- 1 avocado, peeled, pitted and chopped
- 1/2 cup fresh basil, chopped
- 3 garlic cloves, chopped
- 1 tablespoon fresh lemon zest, grated finely

Directions:

1. Grease a large piece of foil.
2. In a large bowl, add all ingredients except salmon and water and with a fork, mash completely.
3. Place fillets in the center of foil and top with avocado mixture evenly.
4. Fold the foil around fillets to seal them.
5. Arrange a steamer trivet in the Instant Pot and pour 1/2 cup of water.

6. Place the foil packet on top of trivet.
7. Close the lid and place the pressure valve to "Seal" position.
8. Press "Manual" and cook under "High Pressure" for about minutes.
9. Meanwhile, preheat the oven to broiler.
10. Press "Cancel" and allow a "Natural" release.
11. Open the lid and transfer the salmon fillets onto a broiler pan.
12. Broil for about 3-4 minutes.
13. Serve warm.

Nutrition Info: Calories 333, Fats 20.3g, Carbs 5.5g, Sugar 0.4g, Proteins 34.2g, Sodium 79mg

Blackened Shrimp

Servings: 4

Cooking Time: 5 Minutes

Ingredients:

- 1 ½ lbs. shrimp, peel & devein
- 4 lime wedges
- 4 tbsp. cilantro, chopped
- What you'll need from store cupboard:
- 4 cloves garlic, diced
- 1 tbsp. chili powder
- 1 tbsp. paprika
- 1 tbsp. olive oil
- 2 tsp Splenda brown sugar
- 1 tsp cumin
- 1 tsp oregano
- 1 tsp garlic powder
- 1 tsp salt
- ½ tsp pepper

Directions:

1.   In a small bowl combine seasonings and Splenda brown sugar.
2.   Heat oil in a skillet over med-high heat. Add shrimp, in a single layer, and cook 1-2 minutes per side.
3.   Add seasonings, and cook, stirring, 30 seconds. Serve garnished with cilantro and a lime wedge.

Nutrition Info: Calories 252 Total Carbs 7g Net Carbs 6g Protein 39g Fat 7g Sugar 2g Fiber 1g

Popcorn Shrimp

Servings: 4

Cooking Time: 8 Minutes

Ingredients:

- Cooking spray
- ½ cup all-purpose flour
- 2 eggs, beaten
- 2 tablespoons water
- 1 ½ cups panko breadcrumbs
- 1 tablespoon garlic powder
- 1 tablespoon ground cumin
- 1 lb. shrimp, peeled and deveined
- ½ cup ketchup
- 2 tablespoons fresh cilantro, chopped
- 2 tablespoons lime juice
- Salt to taste

Directions:

1. Coat the air fryer basket with cooking spray
2. Put the flour in a dish.

3. In the second dish, beat the eggs and water.

4. In the third dish, mix the breadcrumbs, garlic powder and cumin.

5. Dip each shrimp in each of the three dishes, first in the dish with flour, then the egg and then breadcrumb mixture.

6. Place the shrimp in the air fryer basket.

7. Cook at 360 degrees F for 8 minutes, flipping once halfway through.

8. Combine the rest of the ingredients as dipping sauce for the shrimp.

Nutrition Info: Calories 200 g Fat 25 g Carbohydrates 13.8 g Protein 10 g Cholesterol 21 mg

Tuna Carbonara

Servings: 4

Cooking Time: 25 Minutes

Ingredients:

- ½ lb. tuna fillet, cut in pieces
- 2 eggs
- 4 tbsp. fresh parsley, diced
- What you'll need from store cupboard:
- ½ Homemade Pasta, cook & drain, (chapter 15)
- ½ cup reduced fat parmesan cheese
- 2 cloves garlic, peeled
- 2 tbsp. extra virgin olive oil
- Salt & pepper, to taste

Directions:

1. In a small bowl, beat the eggs, parmesan and a dash of pepper.

2. Heat the oil in a large skillet over med-high heat. Add garlic and cook until browned. Add

the tuna and cook 2-3 minutes, or until tuna is almost cooked through. Discard the garlic.

3. Add the pasta and reduce heat. Stir in egg mixture and cook, stirring constantly, 2 minutes. If the sauce is too thick, thin with water, a little bit at a time, until it has a creamy texture.

4. Salt and pepper to taste and serve garnished with parsley.

Nutrition Info: Calories 409 Total Carbs 7g Net Carbs 6g Protein 25g Fat 30g Sugar 3g Fiber 1g

Flavors Cioppino

Servings: 6

Cooking Time: 5 Minutes

Ingredients:

- 1 lb codfish, cut into chunks
- 1 1/2 lbs shrimp
- 28 oz can tomatoes, diced
- 1 cup dry white wine
- 1 bay leaf
- 1 tsp cayenne
- 1 tsp oregano
- 1 shallot, chopped
- 1 tsp garlic, minced
- 1 tbsp olive oil
- 1/2 tsp salt

Directions:

1. Add oil into the inner pot of instant pot and set the pot on sauté mode.
2. Add shallot and garlic and sauté for 2 minutes.
3. Add wine, bay leaf, cayenne, oregano, and salt and cook for 3 minutes.
4. Add remaining ingredients and stir well.
5. Seal pot with a lid and select manual and cook on low for 0 minutes.
6. Once done, release pressure using quick release. Remove lid.
7. Serve and enjoy.

Nutrition Info: Calories 281 Fat 5 g Carbohydrates 10.5 g Sugar 4.9 g Protein 40.7 g Cholesterol 266 mg

Delicious Shrimp Alfredo

Servings: 4

Cooking Time: 3 Minutes

Ingredients:

- 12 shrimp, remove shells
- 1 tbsp garlic, minced
- 1/4 cup parmesan cheese
- 2 cups whole wheat rotini noodles
- 1 cup fish broth
- 15 oz alfredo sauce
- 1 onion, chopped
- Salt

Directions:

1. Add all ingredients except parmesan cheese into the instant pot and stir well.
2. Seal pot with lid and cook on high for 3 minutes.

3. Once done, release pressure using quick release. Remove lid.

4. Stir in cheese and serve.

Nutrition Info: Calories 669 Fat 23.1 g Carbohydrates 76 g Sugar 2.4 g Protein 37.8 g Cholesterol 190 mg

Salmon & Asparagus

Servings: 2

Cooking Time: 10 Minutes

Ingredients:

- 2 salmon fillets

- 8 spears asparagus, trimmed

- 2 tablespoons balsamic vinegar

- 1 teaspoon olive oil

- 1 teaspoon dried dill

- Salt and pepper to taste

Directions:

1. Preheat your oven to 325 degrees F.

2. Dry salmon with paper towels.

3. Arrange the asparagus around the salmon fillets on a baking pan.

4. In a bowl, mix the rest of the ingredients.

5. Pour mixture over the salmon and vegetables.

6.   Bake in the oven for 10 minutes or until the fish is fully cooked.

Nutrition Info: Calories 150 g Fat 22 g Carbohydrates 13.6 g Protein 7 g Cholesterol 20 mg

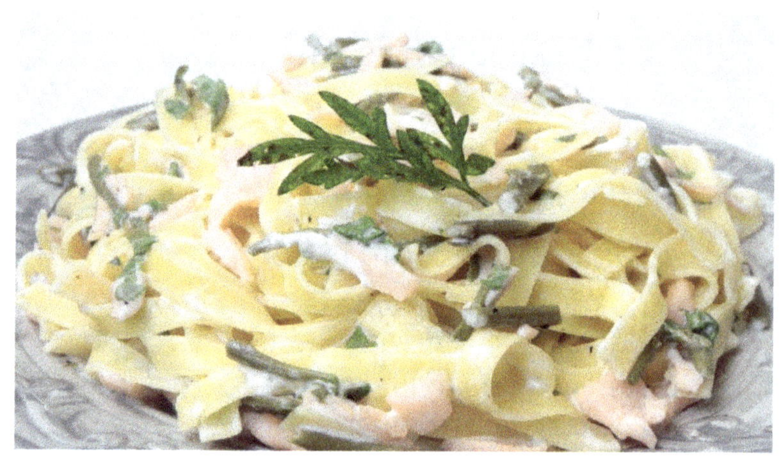

Tuna Sweet Corn Casserole

Servings: 2

Cooking Time: 35 Minutes

Ingredients:

- 3 small tins of tuna

- 0.5lb sweet corn kernels

- 1lb chopped vegetables

- 1 cup low sodium vegetable broth

- 2tbsp spicy seasoning

Directions:

1. Mix all the ingredients in your Instant Pot.

2. Cook on Stew for 35 minutes.

3. Release the pressure naturally.

Nutrition Info: Calories: 300;Carbs: 6 ;Sugar: 1 ;Fat: 9 ;Protein: ;GL: 2

Tortilla Chip With Black Bean Salad

Servings: 4

Cooking Time: 20 Minutes

Ingredients:

- 4 oz. white fish fillets and tortilla chips
- 1/3 cup frozen egg, thawed
- ¼ red onion, chopped
- ¼ teaspoon cumin, ground
- ½ cup cherry tomatoes, halved
- What you will need from the store cupboard:
- 2 teaspoons olive oil
- 1 tablespoon lemon juice
- ¼ teaspoon cayenne pepper
- ½ cup green bell pepper, chopped
- ¼ teaspoon salt
- Cooking spray

Directions:

1. Preheat your oven to 350 ⁰F. Use a foil to line your baking sheet.
2. Apply cooking spray on the foil.
3. Combine the cayenne pepper and tortilla chips in your food processor.
4. Cover till it is crushed fine. Keep in a dish.
5. Use paper towels to pat dry.
6. Pour egg into a second dish. Dip your fish into this and then in your tortilla chips.
7. Now keep the fish on the baking sheet. Coat it with cooking spray lightly.
8. Bake for 8 minutes. The fish must flake easily with a fork.
9. In the meantime, for the salad, bring together the tomatoes, onion, lemon juice, bell pepper, cumin, salt, and oil in your bowl.
10. Place fish on top of the salad. Sprinkle some cheese on top.

Nutrition Info: Calories 361, Carbohydrates 35g, Fiber 8g, Sugar 0.3g, Cholesterol 46mg, Total Fat 11g, Protein 28g

Crunchy Lemon Shrimp

Servings: 4

Cooking Time: 10 Minutes,

Ingredients:

- 1 lb. raw shrimp, peeled and deveined
- 2 tbsp. Italian parsley, roughly chopped
- 2 tbsp. lemon juice, divided
- What you'll need from store cupboard:
- ⅔ cup panko bread crumbs
- 2½ tbsp. olive oil, divided
- Salt and pepper, to taste

Directions:

1. Heat oven to 400 degrees.
2. Place the shrimp evenly in a baking dish and sprinkle with salt and pepper. Drizzle on 1 tablespoon lemon juice and 1 tablespoon of olive oil. Set aside.
3. In a medium bowl, combine parsley, remaining lemon juice, bread crumbs,

remaining olive oil, and ¼ tsp each of salt and pepper. Layer the panko mixture evenly on top of the shrimp.

4. Bake 8-10 minutes or until shrimp are cooked through and the panko is golden brown.

Nutrition Info: Calories 283 Total Carbs 15g Net Carbs 14g Protein 28g Fat 12g Sugar 1g Fiber 1g

Fish Amandine

Servings: 4

Cooking Time: 15 Minutes

Ingredients:

- 4 oz. frozen or fresh tilapia, halibut or trout fillets (skinless, 1-inch size)
- 1/8 teaspoon red pepper, crushed
- ¼ cup almonds, chopped
- ½ cup bread crumbs
- 2 tablespoons parsley, chopped
- What you will need from the store cupboard:
- ½ teaspoon dry mustard
- ¼ cup buttermilk
- 1 tablespoon melted butter
- 2 tablespoons Parmesan cheese, grated
- ¼ teaspoon salt

Directions:

1. Preheat your oven to 350 ºF and grease the baking pan. Keep it aside.
2. Rinse the fish. Use paper towels to pat dry.
3. Now pour the buttermilk into a dish.
4. Take another dish and bring together the parsley, bread crumbs, salt, and dry mustard.
5. Place fish into the buttermilk. Then into your crumb mix.
6. Now keep the coated fish in the baking pan.
7. Sprinkle Parmesan cheese and almonds on the fish. Drizzle melted butter.
8. Also, sprinkle the crushed red pepper.
9. Bake for 4-6 minutes.

Nutrition Info: Calories 209, Carbohydrates 7g, Fiber 1g, Sugar 1g, Cholesterol 67mg, Total Fat 9g, Protein 26g

Shrimp & Veggies Curry

Servings: 6

Cooking Time: 20 Minutes

Ingredients:

- 2 teaspoons olive oil
- 1½ medium white onions, sliced
- 2 medium green bell peppers, seeded and sliced
- 3 medium carrots, peeled and sliced thinly
- 3 garlic cloves, chopped finely
- 1 tablespoon fresh ginger, chopped finely
- 2½ teaspoons curry powder
- 1½ pounds shrimp, peeled and deveined
- 1 cup filtered water
- 2 tablespoons fresh lime juice
- Salt and ground black pepper, as required
- 2 tablespoons fresh cilantro, chopped

Directions:

1. In a large skillet, heat oil over medium-high heat and sauté the onion for about 4-5 minutes.
2. Add the bell peppers and carrot and sauté for about 3-4 minutes.
3. Add the garlic, ginger and curry powder and sauté for about 1 minute.
4. Add the shrimp and sauté for about 1 minute.
5. Stir in the water and cook for about 4-6 minutes, stirring occasionally.
6. Stir in lime juice and remove from heat.
7. Serve hot with the garnishing of cilantro.
8. Meal Prep Tip: Transfer the curry into a large bowl and set aside to cool. Divide the curry into 6 containers evenly. Cover the containers and refrigerate for 1-2 days. Reheat in the microwave before serving.

Nutrition Info: Calories 193 Total Fat 3.8 g Saturated Fat 0.9 g Cholesterol 239 mg Total Carbs 12 g Sugar 4.7 g Fiber 2.3 g Sodium 328 mg Potassium 437 mg Protein 27.1 g

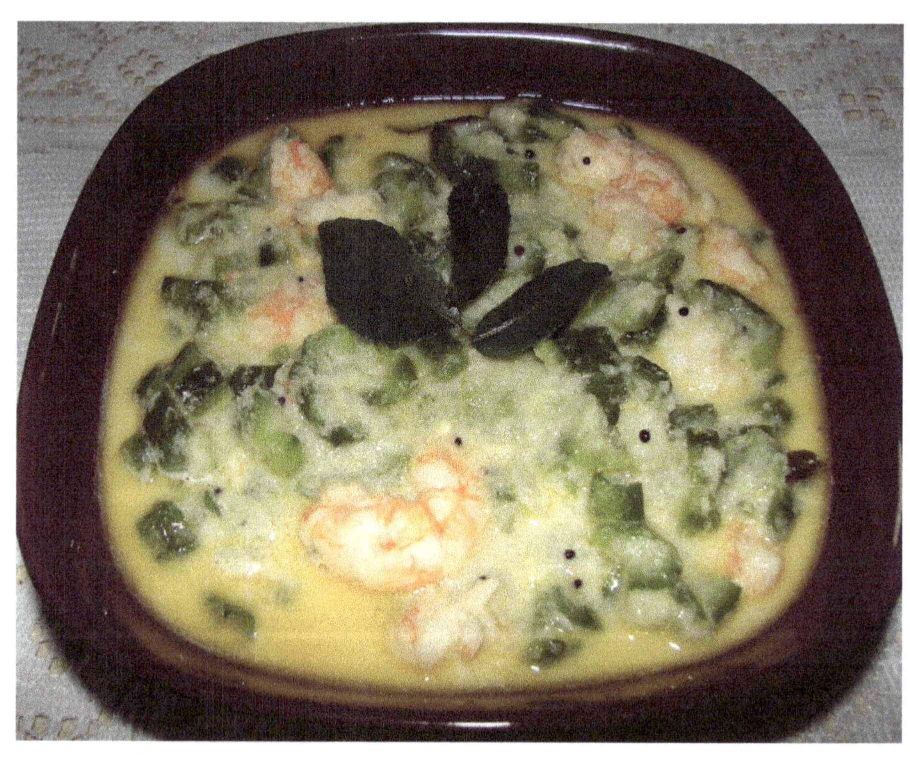

Coconut Clam Chowder

Servings: 6

Cooking Time: 7 Minutes

Ingredients:

- 6 oz clams, chopped
- 1 cup heavy cream
- 1/4 onion, sliced
- 1 cup celery, chopped
- 1 lb cauliflower, chopped
- 1 cup fish broth
- 1 bay leaf
- 2 cups of coconut milk
- Salt

Directions:

1. Add all ingredients except clams and heavy cream and stir well.
2. Seal pot with lid and cook on high for 5 minutes.

3. Once done, release pressure using quick release. Remove lid.

4. Add heavy cream and clams and stir well and cook on sauté mode for 2 minutes.

5. Stir well and serve.

Nutrition Info: Calories 301 Fat 27.2 g Carbohydrates 13.6 g Sugar 6 g Protein 4.9 g Cholesterol 33 mg

Lemon Pepper Salmon

Servings: 4

Cooking Time: 10 Minutes

Ingredients:

- 3 tbsps. ghee or avocado oil
- 1 lb. skin-on salmon filet
- 1 julienned red bell pepper
- 1 julienned green zucchini
- 1 julienned carrot
- ¾ cup water
- A few sprigs of parsley, tarragon, dill, basil or a combination
- 1/2 sliced lemon
- 1/2 tsp. black pepper
- ¼ tsp. sea salt

Directions:

1. Add the water and the herbs into the bottom of the Instant Pot and put in a wire steamer rack making sure the handles extend upwards.
2. Place the salmon filet onto the wire rack, with the skin side facing down.
3. Drizzle the salmon with ghee, season with black pepper and salt, and top with the lemon slices.
4. Close and seal the Instant Pot, making sure the vent is turned to "Sealing".
5. Select the "Steam" setting and cook for 3 minutes.
6. While the salmon cooks, julienne the vegetables, and set aside.
7. Once done, quick release the pressure, and then press the "Keep Warm/Cancel" button.
8. Uncover and wearing oven mitts, carefully remove the steamer rack with the salmon.
9. Remove the herbs and discard them.

10. Add the vegetables to the pot and put the lid back on.

11. Select the "Sauté" function and cook for 1-2 minutes.

12. Serve the vegetables with salmon and add the remaining fat to the pot.

13. Pour a little of the sauce over the fish and vegetables if desired.

Nutrition Info: Calories 296, Carbs 8g, Fat 15 g, Protein 31 g, Potassium (K) 1084 mg, Sodium (Na) 284 mg

Tomato Olive Fish Fillets

Servings: 4

Cooking Time: 8 Minutes

Ingredients:

- 2 lbs halibut fish fillets
- 2 oregano sprigs
- 2 rosemary sprigs
- 2 tbsp fresh lime juice
- 1 cup olives, pitted
- 28 oz can tomatoes, diced
- 1 tbsp garlic, minced
- 1 onion, chopped
- 2 tbsp olive oil

Directions:

1. Add oil into the inner pot of instant pot and set the pot on sauté mode.
2. Add onion and sauté for 3 minutes.
3. Add garlic and sauté for a minute.

4.   Add lime juice, olives, herb sprigs, and tomatoes and stir well.

5.   Seal pot with lid and cook on high for 3 minutes.

6.   Once done, release pressure using quick release. Remove lid.

7.   Add fish fillets and seal pot again with lid and cook on high for 2 minutes.

8.   Once done, release pressure using quick release. Remove lid.

9.   Serve and enjoy.

Nutrition Info: Calories 333 Fat 19.1 g Carbohydrates 31.8 g Sugar 8.4 g Protein 13.4 g Cholesterol 5 mg

Almond Crusted Baked Chili Mahi Mahi

Servings: 4

Cooking Time: 15 Minutes

Ingredients:

- 4 mahi mahi fillets
- 1 lime
- 2 teaspoons olive oil
- Salt and pepper to taste
- ½ cup almonds
- ¼ teaspoon paprika
- ¼ teaspoon onion powder
- ¾ teaspoon chili powder
- ½ cup red bell pepper, chopped
- ¼ cup onion, chopped
- ¼ cup fresh cilantro, chopped

Directions:

1. Preheat your oven to 325 degrees F.
2. Line your baking pan with parchment paper.
3. Squeeze juice from the lime.
4. Grate zest from the peel.
5. Put juice and zest in a bowl.
6. Add the oil, salt and pepper.
7. In another bowl, add the almonds, paprika, onion powder and chili powder.
8. Put the almond mixture in a food processor.
9. Pulse until powdery.
10. Dip each fillet in the oil mixture.
11. Dredge with the almond and chili mixture.
12. Arrange on a single layer in the oven.
13. Bake for 12 to 15 minutes or until fully cooked.
14. Serve with red bell pepper, onion and cilantro.

Nutrition Info: Calories 322 Total Fat 12 g Saturated Fat 2 g Cholesterol 83 mg Sodium 328 mg Total Carbohydrate 28 g Dietary Fiber 4 g Total Sugars 10 g Protein 28 g Potassium 829 mg

Shrimp Lemon Kebab

Servings: 5

Cooking Time: 4 Minutes

Ingredients:

- 1 ½ lb. shrimp, peeled and deveined but with tails intact
- ⅓ cup olive oil
- ¼ cup lemon juice
- 2 teaspoons lemon zest
- 1 tablespoon fresh parsley, chopped
- 8 cherry tomatoes, quartered
- 2 scallions, sliced

Directions:

1. Mix the olive oil, lemon juice, lemon zest and parsley in a bowl.
2. Marinate the shrimp in this mixture for 15 minutes.
3. Thread each shrimp into the skewers.

4. Grill for 4 to 5 minutes, turning once halfway
   through.

5. Serve with tomatoes and scallions.

Nutrition Info: Calories 180 g Fat 20 g
Carbohydrates 15 g Protein 11 g Cholesterol 26 mg

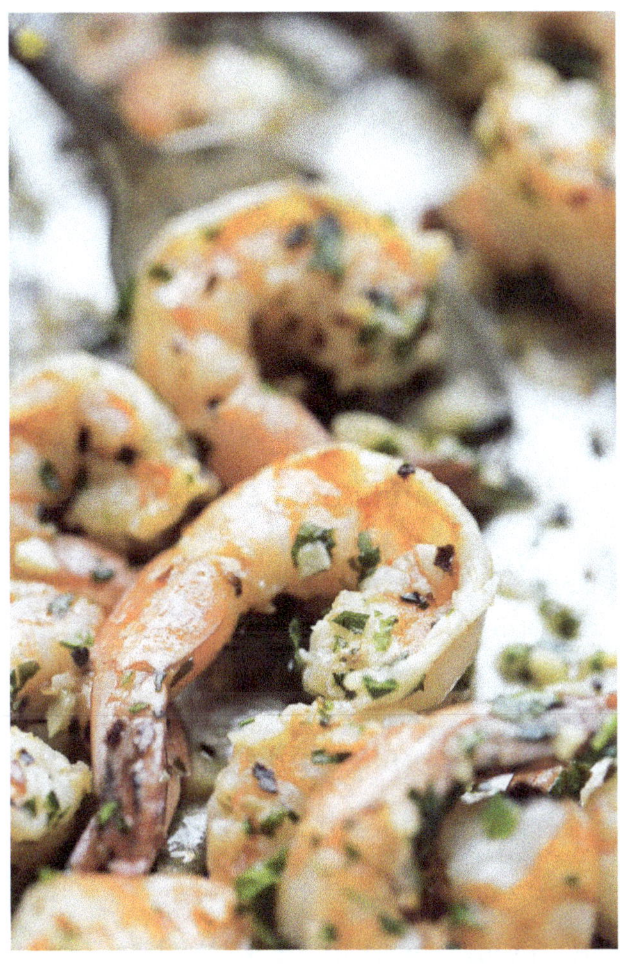

Turkish Tuna With Bulgur And Chickpea Salad

Servings: 4

Cooking Time: 20 Minutes

Ingredients:

- 16 oz. tuna, 4 steaks
- ½ cup bulgur
- 12 oz. chickpeas
- 4 teaspoons lemon zest, grated
- ¼ cup Italian parsley, chopped
- What you will need from the store cupboard:
- ¼ cup extra-virgin olive oil
- ¼ teaspoon ground pepper
- ½ teaspoon salt

Directions:

1. Boil water and keep the bulgur in your bowl.
2. Add 2 inches of the water.

3. Mix your bulgur with 1 tablespoon of oil, pepper, salt, and the lemon zest.

4. Add the chickpeas and parsley.

5. Stir well to combine.

6. Now heat the remaining oil in your skillet over medium heat.

7. Add the tuna. Sear both sides until they become brown.

8. The tuna should flake easily with your fork. Transfer to a plate.

9. In the meantime, bring together ¼ teaspoon salt and the remaining lemon zest in a bowl.

10. Transfer your tuna fish to a serving platter.

11. Sprinkle lemon zest and serve with the bulgur.

Nutrition Info: Calories 459, Carbohydrates 43g, Fiber 8g, Sugar 0.2g, Cholesterol 44mg, Total Fat 16g, Protein 36g

Cajun Flounder & Tomatoes

Servings: 4

Cooking Time: 15 Minutes

Ingredients:

- 4 flounder fillets
- 2 ½ cups tomatoes, diced
- ¾ cup onion, diced
- ¾ cup green bell pepper, diced
- What you'll need from store cupboard:
- 2 cloves garlic, diced fine
- 1 tbsp. Cajun seasoning
- 1 tsp olive oil

Directions:

1. Heat oil in a large skillet over med-high heat. Add onion and garlic and cook 2 minutes, or until soft. Add tomatoes, peppers and spices, and cook 2-3 minutes until tomatoes soften.

2. Lay fish over top. Cover, reduce heat to medium and cook, 5-8 minutes, or until fish

flakes easily with a fork. Transfer fish to serving plates and top with sauce.

Nutrition Info: Calories 194 Total Carbs 8g Net Carbs 6g Protein 32g Fat 3g Sugar 5g Fiber 2g

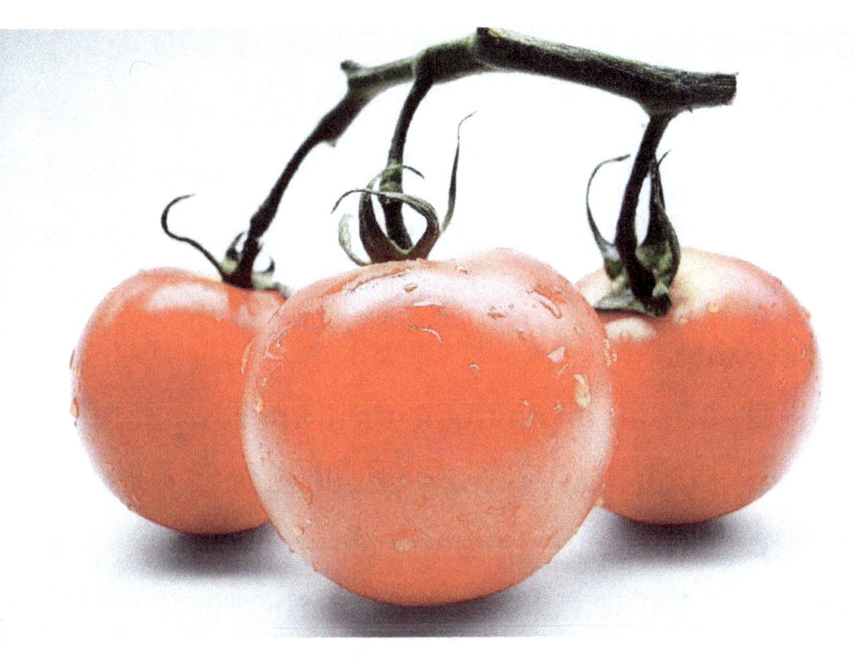

Lemon Sole

Servings: 2

Cooking Time: 5 Minutes

Ingredients:

- 1lb sole fillets, boned and skinned
- 1 cup low sodium fish broth
- 2 shredded sweet onions
- juice of half a lemon
- 2tbsp dried cilantro

Directions:

1. Mix all the ingredients in your Instant Pot.
2. Cook on Stew for 5 minutes.
3. Release the pressure naturally.

Nutrition Info: Calories 230; Carbs Sugar 1; Fat 6; Protein 46; GL 1

Trout Bake

Servings: 2

Cooking Time: 35 Minutes

Ingredients:

- 1lb trout fillets, boneless
- 1lb chopped winter vegetables
- 1 cup low sodium fish broth
- 1tbsp mixed herbs
- sea salt as desired

Directions:

1. Mix all the ingredients except the broth in a foil pouch.
2. Place the pouch in the steamer basket your Instant Pot.
3. Pour the broth into the Instant Pot.
4. Cook on Steam for 35 minutes.
5. Release the pressure naturally.

Nutrition Info: Calories 310; Carbs 14; Sugar 2; Fat 12; Protein 40; GL 5

Garlic Shrimp & Spinach

Servings: 4

Cooking Time: 10 Minutes

Ingredients:

- 3 tablespoons olive oil, divided
- 6 clove garlic, sliced and divided
- 1 lb. spinach
- Salt to taste
- 1 tablespoons lemon juice
- 1 lb. shrimp, peeled and deveined
- ¼ teaspoon red pepper, crushed
- 1 tablespoon parsley, chopped
- 1 teaspoon lemon zest

Directions:

1. Pour 1 tablespoon olive oil in a pot over medium heat.
2. Cook the garlic for 1 minute.
3. Add the spinach and season with salt.
4. Cook for 3 minutes.

5. Stir in lemon juice.

6. Transfer to a bowl.

7. Pour the remaining oil.

8. Add the shrimp.

9. Season with salt and add red pepper.

10. Cook for 5 minutes.

11. Sprinkle parsley and lemon zest over the shrimp before serving.

Nutrition Info: Calories 226 Total Fat 12 g Saturated Fat 2 g Cholesterol 183 mg Sodium 444 mg Total Carbohydrate 6 g Dietary Fiber 3 g Total Sugars 1 g Protein 26 g Potassium 963 mg

Salmon With Bell Peppers

Servings: 6

Cooking Time: 20 Minutes

Ingredients:

- 6 (3-ounce) salmon fillets
- Pinch of salt
- Ground black pepper, as required
- 1 yellow bell pepper, seeded and cubed
- 1 red bell pepper, seeded and cubed
- 4 plum tomatoes, cubed
- 1 small onion, sliced thinly
- ½ cup fresh parsley, chopped
- ¼ cup olive oil
- 2 tablespoons fresh lemon juice

Directions:

1. Preheat the oven to 400 degrees F.
2. Season each salmon fillet with salt and black pepper lightly.

3. In a bowl, mix together the bell peppers, tomato and onion.

4. Arrange 6 foil pieces onto a smooth surface.

5. Place 1 salmon fillet over each foil paper and sprinkle with salt and black pepper.

6. Place veggie mixture over each fillet evenly and top with parsley and capers evenly.

7. Drizzle with oil and lemon juice.

8. Fold each foil around salmon mixture to seal it.

9. Arrange the foil packets onto a large baking sheet in a single layer.

10. Bake for about 20 minutes.

11. Serve hot.

12. Meal Prep Tip: Transfer the salmon mixture into a large bowl and set aside to cool. Divide the salmon mixture into 6 containers evenly. Cover the containers and refrigerate for 1 day. Reheat in the microwave before serving.

Nutrition Info: Calories 220 Total Fat 14 g Saturated Fat 2 g Cholesterol 38 mg Total Carbs 7.7 g Sugar 4.8 g Fiber 2 g Sodium 74 mg Potassium 647 mg Protein 17.9 g

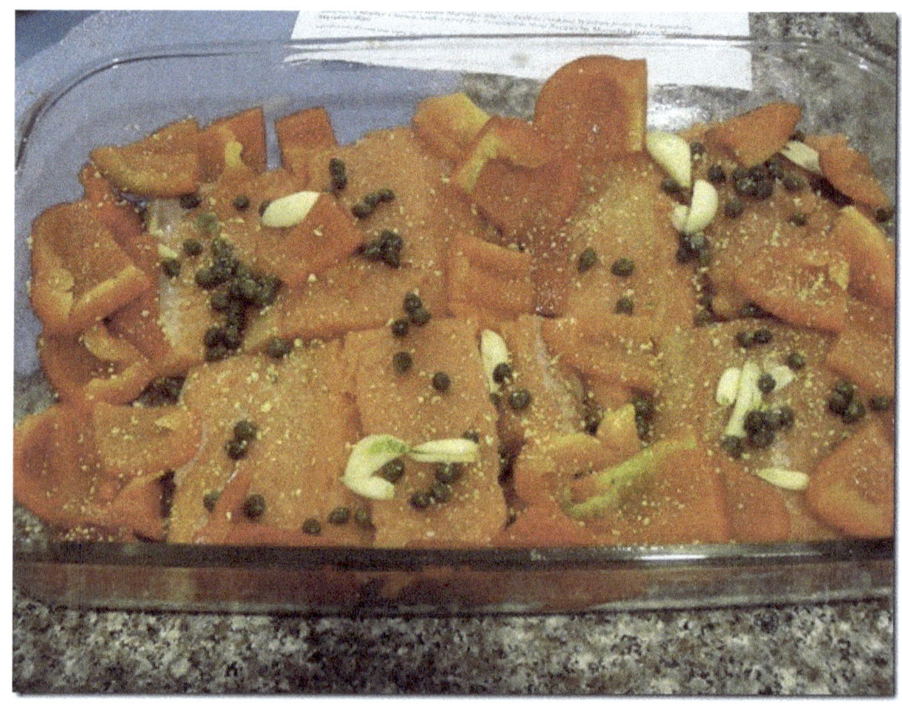

Tarragon Scallops

Servings: 4

Cooking Time: 15 Minutes

Ingredients:

- 1 cup water
- 1 lb. asparagus spears, trimmed
- 2 lemons
- 1 ¼ lb. scallops
- Salt and pepper to taste
- 1 tablespoon olive oil
- 1 tablespoon fresh tarragon, chopped

Directions:

1. Pour water into a pot.
2. Bring to a boil.
3. Add asparagus spears.
4. Cover and cook for 5 minutes.
5. Drain and transfer to a plate.
6. Slice one lemon into wedges.

7. Squeeze juice and shred zest from the remaining lemon.

8. Season the scallops with salt and pepper.

9. Put a pan over medium heat.

10. Add oil to the pan.

11. Cook the scallops until golden brown.

12. Transfer to the same plate, putting scallops beside the asparagus.

13. Add lemon zest, juice and tarragon to the pan.

14. Cook for 1 minute.

15. Drizzle tarragon sauce over the scallops and asparagus.

Nutrition Info: Calories 253 Total Fat 12 g Saturated Fat 2 g Cholesterol 47 mg Sodium 436 mg Total Carbohydrate 14 g Dietary Fiber 5 g Total Sugars 3 g Protein 27 g Potassium 773 mg

Salmon Curry

Servings: 6

Cooking Time: 30 Minutes

Ingredients:

- 6 (4-ounce) salmon fillets
- 1 teaspoon ground turmeric, divided
- Salt, as required
- 3 tablespoon olive oil, divided
- 1 yellow onion, chopped finely
- 1 teaspoon garlic paste
- 1 teaspoon fresh ginger paste
- 3-4 green chilies, halved
- 1 teaspoon red chili powder
- ½ teaspoon ground cumin
- ½ teaspoon ground cinnamon
- ¾ cup fat-free plain Greek yogurt, whipped
- ¾ cup filtered water
- 3 tablespoon fresh cilantro, chopped

Directions:

1. Season each salmon fillet with ½ teaspoon of the turmeric and salt.
2. In a large skillet, melt 1 tablespoon of the butter over medium heat and cook the salmon fillets for about 2 minutes per side.
3. Transfer the salmon onto a plate.
4. In the same skillet, melt the remaining butter over medium heat and sauté the onion for about 4-5 minutes.
5. Add the garlic paste, ginger paste, green chilies, remaining turmeric and spices and sauté for about 1 minute.
6. Now, reduce the heat to medium-low.
7. Slowly, add the yogurt and water, stirring continuously until smooth.
8. Cover the skillet and simmer for about 10-15 minutes or until desired doneness of the sauce.
9. Carefully, add the salmon fillets and simmer for about 5 minutes.
10. Serve hot with the garnishing of cilantro.

11. Meal Prep Tip: Transfer the curry into a large bowl and set aside to cool. Divide the curry into 6 containers evenly. Cover the containers and refrigerate for 1-2 days. Reheat in the microwave before serving.

Nutrition Info: Calories 242 Total Fat 14.3 g Saturated Fat 2 g Cholesterol 51 mg Total Carbs 4.1 g Sugar 2 g Fiber 0.8 g Sodium 98 mg Potassium 493 mg Protein 25.4 g

Halibut With Spicy Apricot Sauce

Servings: 4

Cooking Time: 17 Minutes

Ingredients:

- 4 fresh apricots, pitted
- ⅓ cup apricot preserves
- ½ cup apricot nectar
- ½ teaspoon dried oregano
- 3 tablespoons scallion, sliced
- 1 teaspoon hot pepper sauce
- Salt to taste
- 4 halibut steaks
- 1 tablespoon olive oil

Directions:

1. Put the apricots, preserves, nectar, oregano, scallion, hot pepper sauce and salt in a saucepan.
2. Bring to a boil and then simmer for 8 minutes.

3. Set aside.

4. Brush the halibut steaks with olive oil.

5. Grill for 7 to 9 minutes or until fish is flaky.

6.   Brush one tablespoon of the sauce on both
     sides of the fish.

7. Serve with the reserved sauce.

Nutrition Info: Calories 304 Total Fat 8 g Saturated Fat 1 g Cholesterol 73 mg Sodium 260 mg Total Carbohydrate 27 g Dietary Fiber 2 g Total Sugars 16 g Protein 29 g Potassium 637 mg

Easy Salmon Stew

Servings: 6

Cooking Time: 8 Minutes

Ingredients:

- 2 lbs salmon fillet, cubed
- 1 onion, chopped
- 2 cups fish broth
- 1 tbsp olive oil
- Pepper
- salt

Directions:

1. Add oil into the inner pot of instant pot and set the pot on sauté mode.
2. Add onion and sauté for 2 minutes.
3. Add remaining ingredients and stir well.
4. Seal pot with lid and cook on high for 6 minutes.
5. Once done, release pressure using quick release. Remove lid.

6. Stir and serve.

Nutrition Info: Calories 243 Fat 12.6 g Carbohydrates 0.8 g Sugar 0.3 g Protein 31 g Cholesterol 78 mg

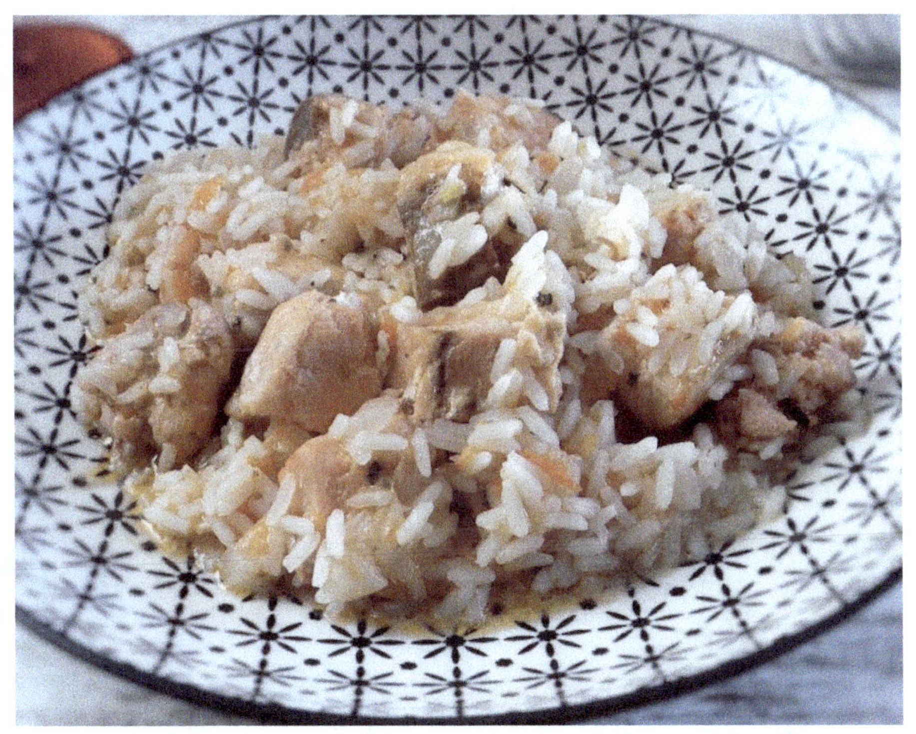

Cilantro Lime Grilled Shrimp

Servings: 6

Cooking Time: 5 Minutes,

Ingredients:

- 1 ½ lbs. large shrimp raw, peeled, deveined with tails on
- Juice and zest of 1 lime
- 2 tbsp. fresh cilantro chopped
- What you'll need from store cupboard:
- ¼ cup olive oil
- 2 cloves garlic, diced fine
- 1 tsp smoked paprika
- ¼ tsp cumin
- 1/2 teaspoon salt
- ¼ tsp cayenne pepper

Directions:

1. Place the shrimp in a large Ziploc bag.

2. Mix remaining Ingredients in a small bowl and pour over shrimp. Let marinate 20-30 minutes.

3. Heat up the grill. Skewer the shrimp and cook 2-3 minutes, per side, just until they turn pick. Be careful not to overcook them. Serve garnished with cilantro.

Nutrition Info: Calories 317 Total Carbs 4g Protein 39g Fat 15g Sugar 0g Fiber 0g

Cajun Catfish

Servings: 4

Cooking Time: 15 Minutes

Ingredients:

- 4 (8 oz.) catfish fillets
- What you'll need from store cupboard:
- 2 tbsp. olive oil
- 2 tsp garlic salt
- 2 tsp thyme
- 2 tsp paprika
- ½ tsp cayenne pepper
- ½ tsp red hot sauce
- ¼ tsp black pepper
- Nonstick cooking spray

Directions:

1. Heat oven to 450 degrees. Spray a 9x13-inch baking dish with cooking spray.
2. In a small bowl whisk together everything but catfish. Brush both sides of fillets, using all the spice mix.
3. Bake 10-13 minutes or until fish flakes easily with a fork. Serve.

Nutrition Info: Calories 366 Total Carbs 0g Protein 35g Fat 24g Sugar 0g Fiber 0g

Halibut With Spicy Apricot Sauce

Servings: 4

Cooking Time: 17 Minutes

Ingredients:

- 4 fresh apricots, pitted
- ⅓ cup apricot preserves
- ½ cup apricot nectar
- ½ teaspoon dried oregano
- 3 tablespoons scallion, sliced
- 1 teaspoon hot pepper sauce
- Salt to taste
- 4 halibut steaks
- 1 tablespoon olive oil

Directions:

1. Put the apricots, preserves, nectar, oregano, scallion, hot pepper sauce and salt in a saucepan.
2. Bring to a boil and then simmer for 8 minutes.
3. Set aside.
4. Brush the halibut steaks with olive oil.
5. Grill for 7 to 9 minutes or until fish is flaky.
6. Brush one tablespoon of the sauce on both sides of the fish.
7. Serve with the reserved sauce.
8. Bake in the oven for 10 minutes or until the fish is fully cooked.

Nutrition Info: Calories 150 g Fat 22 g Carbohydrates 13.6 g Protein 7 g Cholesterol 20 mg

Mixed Chowder

Servings: 2

Cooking Time: 35 Minutes

Ingredients:

- 1lb fish stew mix
- 2 cups white sauce
- 3tbsp old bay seasoning

Directions:

1. Mix all the ingredients in your Instant Pot.
2. Cook on Stew for 35 minutes.
3. Release the pressure naturally.

Nutrition Info: Calories 320; Carbs 9; Sugar 2; Fat 16; Protein GL 4

Shrimp With Zucchini

Servings: 4

Cooking Time: 8 Minutes

Ingredients:

- 3 tablespoons olive oil
- 1 pound medium shrimp, peeled and deveined
- 1 shallot, minced
- 4 garlic cloves, minced
- ¼ teaspoon red pepper flakes, crushed
- Salt and ground black pepper, as required
- ¼ cup low-sodium chicken broth
- 2 tablespoons fresh lemon juice
- 1 teaspoon fresh lemon zest, grated finely
- ½ pound zucchini, spiralized with Blade C

Directions:

1. In a large skillet, heat the oil and butter over medium-high heat and cook the shrimp, shallot, garlic, red pepper flakes, salt and

black pepper for about 2 minutes, stirring occasionally.

2. Stir in the broth, lemon juice and lemon zest and bring to a gentle boil.

3. Stir in zucchini noodles and cook for about 1-2 minutes.

4. Serve hot.

5. Meal Prep Tip: Transfer the shrimp mixture into a large bowl and set aside to cool. Divide the shrimp mixture into 4 containers. Cover the containers and refrigerate for about 1-2 days. Reheat in microwave before serving.

Nutrition Info: Calories 245 Total Fat 12.6 g Saturated Fat 2.2 g Cholesterol 239 mg Total Carbs 5.8 g Sugar 1.2 g Fiber 08 g Sodium 289 mg Potassium 381 mg Protein 27 g

Braised Shrimp

Servings: 4

Cooking Time: 4 Minutes

Ingredients:

- 1 pound frozen large shrimp, peeled and deveined
- 2 shallots, chopped
- ¾ cup low-sodium chicken broth
- 2 tablespoons fresh lemon juice
- 2 tablespoons olive oil
- 1 tablespoon garlic, crushed
- Ground black pepper, as required

Directions:

1. In the Instant Pot, place oil and press "Sauté". Now add the shallots and cook for about 2 minutes.
2. Add the garlic and cook for about 1 minute.
3. Press "Cancel" and stir in the shrimp, broth, lemon juice and black pepper.

4.   Close the lid and place the pressure valve to "Seal" position.

5.   Press "Manual" and cook under "High Pressure" for about 1 minute.

6.   Press "Cancel" and carefully allow a "Quick" release.

7.   Open the lid and serve hot.

Nutrition Info: Calories 209, Fats 9g, Carbs 4.3g, Sugar 0.2g, Proteins 26.6g, Sodium 293mg

Salmon Soup

Servings: 4

Cooking Time: 20 Minutes

Ingredients:

- 1 tablespoon olive oil
- 1 yellow onion, chopped
- 1 garlic clove, minced
- 4 cups low-sodium chicken broth
- 1 pound boneless salmon, cubed
- 2 tablespoon fresh cilantro, chopped
- Ground black pepper, as required
- 1 tablespoon fresh lime juice

Directions:

1. In a large pan heat the oil over medium heat and sauté the onion for about 5 minutes.
2. Add the garlic and sauté for about 1 minute.
3. Stir in the broth and bring to a boil over high heat.

4. Now, reduce the heat to low and simmer for about 10 minutes.

5. Add the salmon, and soy sauce and cook for about 3-4 minutes.

6. Stir in black pepper, lime juice, and cilantro and serve hot.

7. Meal Prep Tip: Transfer the soup into a large bowl and set aside to cool. Divide the soup into 4 containers evenly. Cover the containers and refrigerate for 1-2 days. Reheat in the microwave before serving.

Nutrition Info: Calories 208 Total Fat 10.5 g Saturated Fat 1.5 g Cholesterol 50 mg Total Carbs 3.9 g Sugar 1.2 g Fiber 0.6 g Sodium 121 mg Potassium 331 mg Protein 24.4

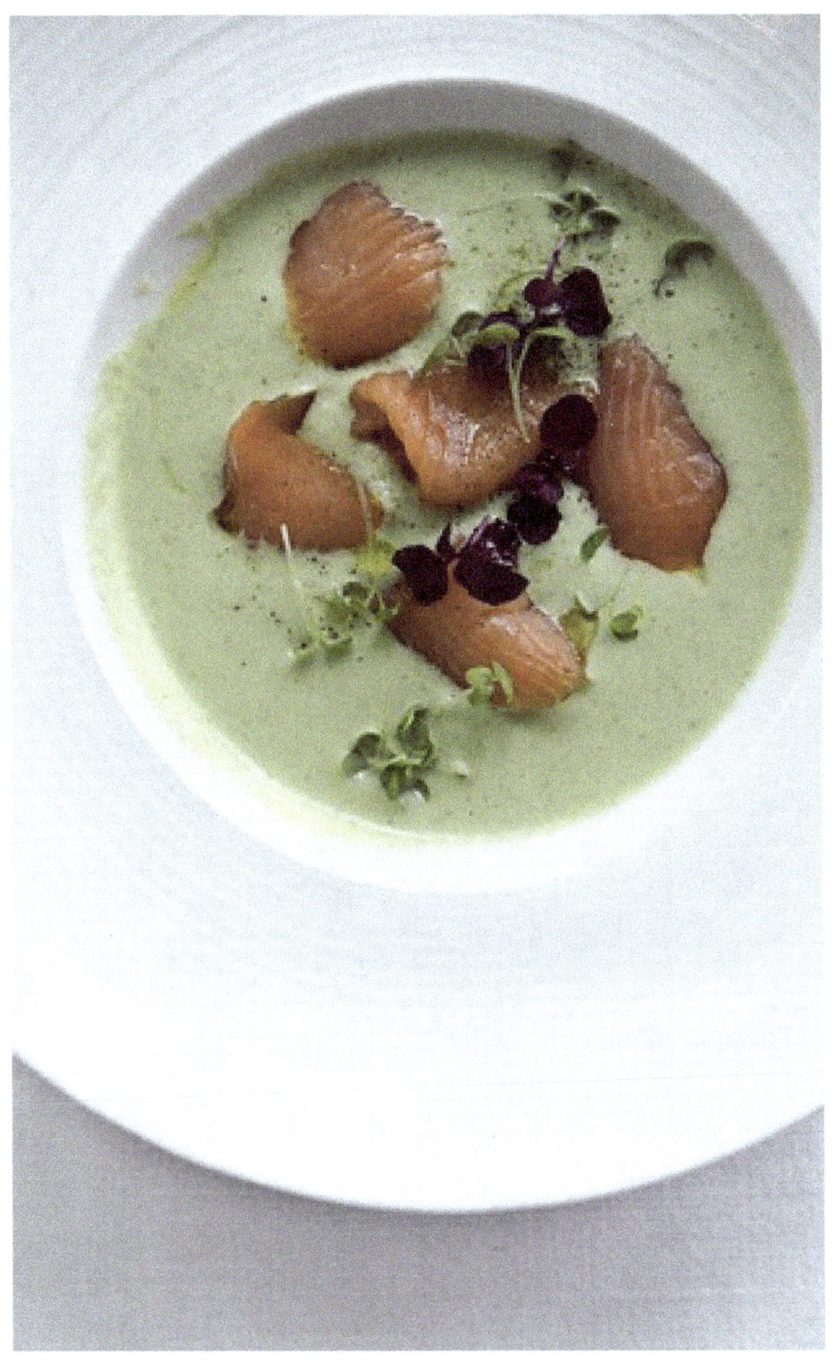

www.ingramcontent.com/pod-product-compliance
Lightning Source LLC
Chambersburg PA
CBHW061000050726
47592CB00003B/1283